This journal belongs to

_____

Training
FOR A
Healthy
Life

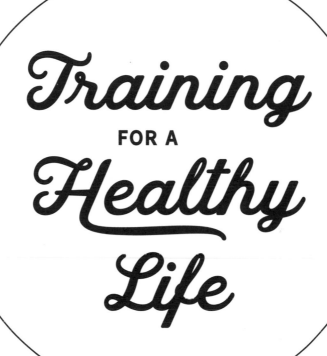

Training
FOR A
Healthy
Life

A DAILY FOOD
& FITNESS JOURNAL

Published in the United States by Zeitgeist Wellness, an imprint of Zeitgeist™, a division of Penguin Random House LLC, New York.
penguinrandomhouse.com

Zeitgeist™ is a trademark of Penguin Random House LLC
ISBN: 9780593196595

Illustrations © Shirstok/Shutterstock.com
Book design by Katy Brown

Printed in the United States of America
  7 9 10 8

First Edition

To you,
for taking control of your diet,
exercise, and health.

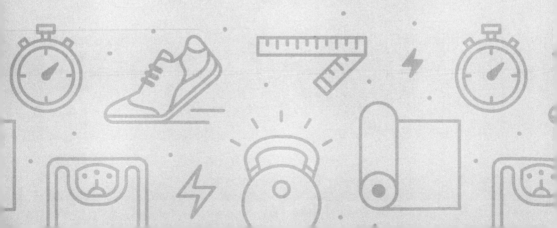

"Some people want it to happen, some wish it would happen, others make it happen."

—MICHAEL JORDAN, SIX-TIME NBA CHAMPION

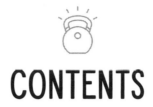

CONTENTS

LET'S START TRAINING!

Congratulations on starting your journey to a healthy, new you! By recording your food, exercise, and wellness details along with your goals, you are well on your way to better health.

This journal is easy to use: you'll begin by recording your current weight and measurements, then jotting down the goals you hope to achieve by the end of 13 weeks.

Every day you'll record your weight, your daily goal, what you ate, how much you exercised, and how well you took care of yourself. At the end of each week you'll have the chance to review the previous seven days and chart your progress. When you've completed your journal you'll be able to note your new weight and measurements, and look back on how much progress you made. You'll even have space to record new goals going forward.

On page 4, you'll find a completed daily activity page with ideas for how to use this book. But you should feel free to fill out this journal any way you want: it's your journal and your journey. Do whatever you want to make it yours!

In 13 weeks you'll solidify healthy new habits and notice the difference these habits are making on you. Your daily records will keep you focused on your goals, giving you a greater chance of meeting them. So turn the page, start writing, and begin training for a healthy life!

YOUR STARTING POINT

You can only track your progress if you know where you're starting from. Record your weight and measurements here (and anything else you want to track), and refer back to these numbers weekly, monthly, or at the end of your journey—or at all points along the way.

DATE:_____   WEIGHT:_____

MEASUREMENTS

CHEST	
WAIST	
HIPS	
THIGHS	
CALVES	
UPPER ARMS	

OTHER STATS TO TRACK

_____

_____

_____

_____

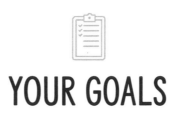

YOUR GOALS

WEIGHT: _____

MEASUREMENTS

CHEST	
WAIST	
HIPS	
THIGHS	
CALVES	
UPPER ARMS	

OTHER STATS

A SAMPLE DAY

DATE: 10/17   WEIGHT: 150

GOAL FOR TODAY
get back into regular gym routine

FOOD

BREAKFAST	eggs
LUNCH	turkey sandwich
DINNER	roast chicken and vegetables
SNACKS	almonds

EXERCISE

TYPE OF EXERCISE	AMOUNT	NOTES
cardio - treadmill	20 minutes	incline = 3
weights	30 minutes	focus on arms

WELLNESS

I DRANK _____ 8 _____ [(CUPS) / BOTTLES / OUNCES] OF WATER.

I SLEPT _____ 8 _____ HOURS.

MY MOOD IS *stressed*

I TOOK CARE OF MYSELF BY *hitting it hard at the gym*

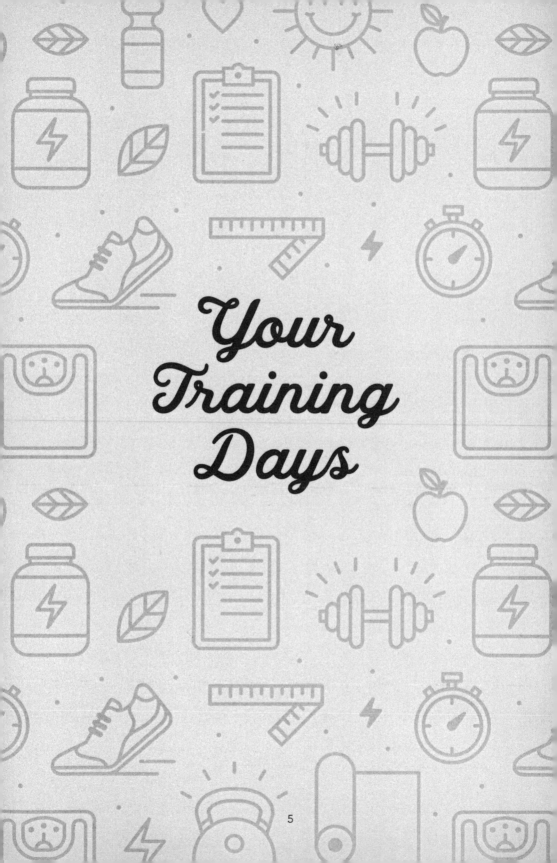

Your Training Days

DATE: _____   WEIGHT: _____

GOAL FOR TODAY

_____

_____

_____

🍎 FOOD

BREAKFAST	
LUNCH	
DINNER	
SNACKS	

EXERCISE

TYPE OF EXERCISE	AMOUNT	NOTES

❤ WELLNESS

I DRANK _____ [CUPS / BOTTLES / OUNCES] OF WATER.

I SLEPT _____ HOURS.

MY MOOD IS _____

_____

I TOOK CARE OF MYSELF BY _____

_____

DATE: _____   WEIGHT: _____

GOAL FOR TODAY

_____
_____
_____

FOOD

BREAKFAST	_____
LUNCH	_____
DINNER	_____
SNACKS	_____

EXERCISE

TYPE OF EXERCISE	AMOUNT	NOTES

WELLNESS

I DRANK _____ [CUPS / BOTTLES / OUNCES] OF WATER.

I SLEPT _____ HOURS.

MY MOOD IS _____
_____

I TOOK CARE OF MYSELF BY _____
_____

DATE: _____   WEIGHT: _____

GOAL FOR TODAY

_____

_____

_____

🍎 FOOD

BREAKFAST	
LUNCH	
DINNER	
SNACKS	

🏋 EXERCISE

TYPE OF EXERCISE	AMOUNT	NOTES

♥ WELLNESS

I DRANK _____ [CUPS / BOTTLES / OUNCES] OF WATER.

I SLEPT _____ HOURS.

MY MOOD IS

_____

_____

I TOOK CARE OF MYSELF BY

_____

_____

DATE: _____   WEIGHT: _____

GOAL FOR TODAY

_____

_____

_____

🍎 FOOD

BREAKFAST	
LUNCH	
DINNER	
SNACKS	

🏋 EXERCISE

TYPE OF EXERCISE	AMOUNT	NOTES

♥ WELLNESS

I DRANK _____ [CUPS / BOTTLES / OUNCES] OF WATER.

I SLEPT _____ HOURS.

MY MOOD IS _____

_____

I TOOK CARE OF MYSELF BY _____

_____

DATE: _____   WEIGHT: _____

GOAL FOR TODAY

_____

_____

_____

🍎 FOOD

BREAKFAST	
LUNCH	
DINNER	
SNACKS	

🏋 EXERCISE

TYPE OF EXERCISE	AMOUNT	NOTES

❤ WELLNESS

I DRANK _____ [CUPS / BOTTLES / OUNCES] OF WATER.

I SLEPT _____ HOURS.

MY MOOD IS _____

_____

I TOOK CARE OF MYSELF BY _____

_____

DATE: _____   WEIGHT: _____

GOAL FOR TODAY

_____

_____

_____

_____

FOOD

BREAKFAST	
LUNCH	
DINNER	
SNACKS	

EXERCISE

TYPE OF EXERCISE	AMOUNT	NOTES

WELLNESS

I DRANK _____ [CUPS / BOTTLES / OUNCES] OF WATER.

I SLEPT _____ HOURS.

MY MOOD IS _____

_____

I TOOK CARE OF MYSELF BY _____

_____

DATE: _____   WEIGHT: _____

GOAL FOR TODAY

_____

_____

_____

FOOD

BREAKFAST	
LUNCH	
DINNER	
SNACKS	

EXERCISE

TYPE OF EXERCISE	AMOUNT	NOTES

WELLNESS

I DRANK _____ [CUPS / BOTTLES / OUNCES] OF WATER.

I SLEPT _____ HOURS.

MY MOOD IS _____

_____

I TOOK CARE OF MYSELF BY _____

_____

Weekly Check-In

Here's your chance to review your progress over the last seven days.

DATE: _____   WEIGHT: _____

MEASUREMENTS

CHEST		THIGHS	
WAIST		CALVES	
HIPS		UPPER ARMS	

OTHER STATS

_____

_____

_____

_____

Are you satisfied with how you did this week in the following areas?
Do you see room for improvement? How?

FOOD
_____

EXERCISE
_____

WATER
_____

SLEEP
_____

SELF-CARE
_____

DATE: _____   WEIGHT: _____

GOAL FOR TODAY

_____

_____

_____

FOOD

BREAKFAST	
LUNCH	
DINNER	
SNACKS	

EXERCISE

TYPE OF EXERCISE	AMOUNT	NOTES

WELLNESS

I DRANK _____ [CUPS / BOTTLES / OUNCES] OF WATER.

I SLEPT _____ HOURS.

MY MOOD IS

_____

_____

I TOOK CARE OF MYSELF BY

_____

DATE: _____ WEIGHT: _____

GOAL FOR TODAY

_____

_____

_____

FOOD

BREAKFAST°	
LUNCH	
DINNER	
SNACKS	

EXERCISE

TYPE OF EXERCISE	AMOUNT	NOTES

WELLNESS

I DRANK _____ [CUPS / BOTTLES / OUNCES] OF WATER.

I SLEPT _____ HOURS.

MY MOOD IS _____

_____

I TOOK CARE OF MYSELF BY _____

_____

DATE: _____   WEIGHT: _____

GOAL FOR TODAY

_____

_____

_____

FOOD

BREAKFAST	
LUNCH	
DINNER	
SNACKS	

EXERCISE

TYPE OF EXERCISE	AMOUNT	NOTES

WELLNESS

I DRANK _____ [CUPS / BOTTLES / OUNCES] OF WATER.

I SLEPT _____ HOURS.

MY MOOD IS
_____

_____

I TOOK CARE OF MYSELF BY
_____

_____

DATE: _____   WEIGHT: _____

GOAL FOR TODAY

_____

_____

_____

FOOD

BREAKFAST	
LUNCH	
DINNER	
SNACKS	

EXERCISE

TYPE OF EXERCISE	AMOUNT	NOTES

WELLNESS

I DRANK _____ [CUPS / BOTTLES / OUNCES] OF WATER.

I SLEPT _____ HOURS.

MY MOOD IS _____

_____

I TOOK CARE OF MYSELF BY _____

_____

DATE: _____   WEIGHT: _____

GOAL FOR TODAY

_____

_____

_____

FOOD

BREAKFAST	
LUNCH	
DINNER	
SNACKS	

EXERCISE

TYPE OF EXERCISE	AMOUNT	NOTES

WELLNESS

I DRANK _____ [CUPS / BOTTLES / OUNCES] OF WATER.

I SLEPT _____ HOURS.

MY MOOD IS _____

_____

I TOOK CARE OF MYSELF BY _____

_____

DATE: _____   WEIGHT: _____

GOAL FOR TODAY

_____

_____

_____

🍎 FOOD

BREAKFAST	
LUNCH	
DINNER	
SNACKS	

EXERCISE

TYPE OF EXERCISE	AMOUNT	NOTES

♥ WELLNESS

I DRANK _____ [CUPS / BOTTLES / OUNCES] OF WATER.

I SLEPT _____ HOURS.

MY MOOD IS _____

_____

I TOOK CARE OF MYSELF BY _____

_____

DATE: _____   WEIGHT: _____

GOAL FOR TODAY

_____
_____
_____

FOOD

BREAKFAST	
LUNCH	
DINNER	
SNACKS ·	

EXERCISE

TYPE OF EXERCISE	AMOUNT	NOTES

WELLNESS

I DRANK _____ [CUPS / BOTTLES / OUNCES] OF WATER.

I SLEPT _____ HOURS.

MY MOOD IS _____
_____

I TOOK CARE OF MYSELF BY _____
_____

Weekly Check-In

Here's your chance to review your progress over the last seven days.

DATE: _____   WEIGHT: _____

MEASUREMENTS

CHEST		THIGHS	
WAIST		CALVES	
HIPS		UPPER ARMS	

OTHER STATS

_____

_____

_____

_____

Are you satisfied with how you did this week in the following areas?
Do you see room for improvement? How?

FOOD
_____

_____

EXERCISE
_____

_____

WATER
_____

SLEEP
_____

SELF-CARE
_____

_____

DATE: _____ -   WEIGHT: _____

GOAL FOR TODAY

_____

_____

_____

FOOD

BREAKFAST	
LUNCH	
DINNER	
SNACKS	

EXERCISE

TYPE OF EXERCISE	AMOUNT	NOTES

WELLNESS

I DRANK _____ [CUPS / BOTTLES / OUNCES] OF WATER.

I SLEPT _____ HOURS.

MY MOOD IS _____

_____

I TOOK CARE OF MYSELF BY _____

_____

DATE: _____   WEIGHT: _____

GOAL FOR TODAY

_____

_____

_____

FOOD

BREAKFAST	
LUNCH	
DINNER	
SNACKS	

EXERCISE

TYPE OF EXERCISE	AMOUNT	NOTES

WELLNESS

I DRANK _____ [CUPS / BOTTLES / OUNCES] OF WATER.

I SLEPT _____ HOURS.

MY MOOD IS _____

_____

I TOOK CARE OF MYSELF BY _____

_____

DATE: _____   WEIGHT: _____

GOAL FOR TODAY

_____

_____

_____

FOOD

BREAKFAST	
LUNCH	
DINNER	
SNACKS	

EXERCISE

TYPE OF EXERCISE	AMOUNT	NOTES

WELLNESS

I DRANK _____ [CUPS / BOTTLES / OUNCES] OF WATER.

I SLEPT _____ HOURS.

MY MOOD IS _____

_____

I TOOK CARE OF MYSELF BY _____

_____

DATE: _____   WEIGHT: _____

GOAL FOR TODAY

_____

_____

_____

🍎 FOOD

BREAKFAST	
LUNCH	
DINNER	
SNACKS	

🏋 EXERCISE

TYPE OF EXERCISE	AMOUNT	NOTES

💗 WELLNESS

I DRANK _____ [CUPS / BOTTLES / OUNCES] OF WATER.

I SLEPT _____ HOURS.

MY MOOD IS _____

_____

I TOOK CARE OF MYSELF BY _____

_____

DATE: _____   WEIGHT: _____

GOAL FOR TODAY

_____

_____

_____

FOOD

BREAKFAST	
LUNCH	
DINNER	
SNACKS	

EXERCISE

TYPE OF EXERCISE	AMOUNT	NOTES

WELLNESS

I DRANK _____ [CUPS / BOTTLES / OUNCES] OF WATER.

I SLEPT _____ HOURS.

MY MOOD IS

_____

I TOOK CARE OF MYSELF BY

_____

DATE: _____   WEIGHT: _____

GOAL FOR TODAY

_____

_____

_____

🍎 FOOD

BREAKFAST	
LUNCH	
DINNER	
SNACKS	

🏋 EXERCISE

TYPE OF EXERCISE	AMOUNT	NOTES

❤ WELLNESS

I DRANK _____ [CUPS / BOTTLES / OUNCES] OF WATER.

I SLEPT _____ HOURS.

MY MOOD IS _____

_____

I TOOK CARE OF MYSELF BY _____

_____

DATE: _____   WEIGHT: _____

GOAL FOR TODAY

_____
_____
_____

FOOD

BREAKFAST	
LUNCH	
DINNER	
SNACKS	

EXERCISE

TYPE OF EXERCISE	AMOUNT	NOTES

WELLNESS

I DRANK _____ [CUPS / BOTTLES / OUNCES] OF WATER.

I SLEPT _____ HOURS.

MY MOOD IS
_____
_____

I TOOK CARE OF MYSELF BY
_____
_____

Weekly Check-In

Here's your chance to review your progress over the last seven days.

DATE: _____ WEIGHT: _____

MEASUREMENTS

CHEST		THIGHS	
WAIST		CALVES	
HIPS		UPPER ARMS	

OTHER STATS

_____

_____

_____

_____

Are you satisfied with how you did this week in the following areas?
Do you see room for improvement? How?

FOOD
_____

EXERCISE
_____

WATER
_____

SLEEP
_____

SELF-CARE
_____

DATE: _____   WEIGHT: _____

GOAL FOR TODAY

_____
_____
_____

FOOD

BREAKFAST	
LUNCH	
DINNER	
SNACKS	

EXERCISE

TYPE OF EXERCISE	AMOUNT	NOTES

WELLNESS

I DRANK _____ [CUPS / BOTTLES / OUNCES] OF WATER.

I SLEPT _____ HOURS.

MY MOOD IS _____

_____

I TOOK CARE OF MYSELF BY _____

_____

DATE: _____   WEIGHT: _____

GOAL FOR TODAY

_____

_____

_____

🍎 FOOD

BREAKFAST	
LUNCH	
DINNER	
SNACKS	

🏋 EXERCISE

TYPE OF EXERCISE	AMOUNT	NOTES

♥ WELLNESS

I DRANK _____ [CUPS / BOTTLES / OUNCES] OF WATER.

I SLEPT _____ HOURS.

MY MOOD IS _____

_____

I TOOK CARE OF MYSELF BY _____

_____

DATE: _____ WEIGHT: _____

GOAL FOR TODAY

_____
_____
_____

FOOD

BREAKFAST	
LUNCH	
DINNER	
SNACKS	

EXERCISE

TYPE OF EXERCISE	AMOUNT	NOTES

WELLNESS

I DRANK _____ [CUPS / BOTTLES / OUNCES] OF WATER.

I SLEPT _____ HOURS.

MY MOOD IS _____
_____

I TOOK CARE OF MYSELF BY _____
_____

DATE: _____   WEIGHT: _____

GOAL FOR TODAY

_____

_____

_____

🍎 FOOD

BREAKFAST	
LUNCH	
DINNER	
SNACKS	

🏋 EXERCISE

TYPE OF EXERCISE	AMOUNT	NOTES

❤ WELLNESS

I DRANK _____ [CUPS / BOTTLES / OUNCES] OF WATER.

I SLEPT _____ HOURS.

MY MOOD IS _____

_____

I TOOK CARE OF MYSELF BY _____

_____

DATE: _____   WEIGHT: _____

GOAL FOR TODAY

_____
_____
_____

FOOD

BREAKFAST	
LUNCH	
DINNER	
SNACKS	

EXERCISE

TYPE OF EXERCISE	AMOUNT	NOTES

WELLNESS

I DRANK _____ [CUPS / BOTTLES / OUNCES] OF WATER.

I SLEPT _____ HOURS.

MY MOOD IS _____

_____

I TOOK CARE OF MYSELF BY _____

_____

DATE: _____   WEIGHT: _____

GOAL FOR TODAY

_____

_____

_____

FOOD

BREAKFAST	
LUNCH	
DINNER	
SNACKS	

EXERCISE

TYPE OF EXERCISE	AMOUNT	NOTES

WELLNESS

I DRANK _____ [CUPS / BOTTLES / OUNCES] OF WATER.

I SLEPT _____ HOURS.

MY MOOD IS _____

_____

I TOOK CARE OF MYSELF BY _____

_____

DATE: _____ WEIGHT: _____

GOAL FOR TODAY

_____
_____
_____

FOOD

BREAKFAST	
LUNCH	
DINNER	
SNACKS	

EXERCISE

TYPE OF EXERCISE	AMOUNT	NOTES

WELLNESS

I DRANK _____ [CUPS / BOTTLES / OUNCES] OF WATER.

I SLEPT _____ HOURS.

MY MOOD IS _____
_____

I TOOK CARE OF MYSELF BY _____ .
_____

Weekly Check-In

Here's your chance to review your progress over the last seven days.

DATE: _____   WEIGHT: _____

✎ MEASUREMENTS

CHEST		THIGHS	
WAIST		CALVES	
HIPS		UPPER ARMS	

📋 OTHER STATS

_____

_____

_____

_____

Are you satisfied with how you did this week in the following areas? Do you see room for improvement? How?

FOOD
_____

EXERCISE
_____

WATER
_____

SLEEP
_____

SELF-CARE
_____

DATE: _____   WEIGHT: _____

GOAL FOR TODAY

_____

_____

_____

FOOD

BREAKFAST	
LUNCH	
DINNER	
SNACKS	

EXERCISE

TYPE OF EXERCISE	AMOUNT	NOTES

WELLNESS

I DRANK _____ [CUPS / BOTTLES / OUNCES] OF WATER.

I SLEPT _____ HOURS.

MY MOOD IS _____

_____

I TOOK CARE OF MYSELF BY _____

_____

DATE: _____   WEIGHT: _____

GOAL FOR TODAY

_____
_____
_____
_____

🍎 FOOD

BREAKFAST	
LUNCH	
DINNER	
SNACKS .	

🏋 EXERCISE

TYPE OF EXERCISE	AMOUNT	NOTES

♥ WELLNESS

I DRANK _____ [CUPS / BOTTLES / OUNCES] OF WATER.

I SLEPT _____ HOURS.

MY MOOD IS _____
_____

I TOOK CARE OF MYSELF BY _____
_____

DATE: _____   WEIGHT: _____

GOAL FOR TODAY

_____

_____

_____

🍎 FOOD

BREAKFAST	
LUNCH	
DINNER	
SNACKS	

🏋 EXERCISE

TYPE OF EXERCISE	AMOUNT	NOTES

♥ WELLNESS

I DRANK _____ [CUPS / BOTTLES / OUNCES] OF WATER.

I SLEPT _____ HOURS.

MY MOOD IS

_____

_____

I TOOK CARE OF MYSELF BY

_____

DATE: _____   WEIGHT: _____

GOAL FOR TODAY

_____

_____

_____

_____

FOOD

BREAKFAST	
LUNCH	
DINNER	
SNACKS	

EXERCISE

TYPE OF EXERCISE	AMOUNT	NOTES

WELLNESS

I DRANK _____ [CUPS / BOTTLES / OUNCES] OF WATER.

I SLEPT _____ HOURS.

MY MOOD IS _____

_____

I TOOK CARE OF MYSELF BY _____

_____

DATE: _____   WEIGHT: _____

GOAL FOR TODAY

_____

_____

_____

🍎 FOOD

BREAKFAST	
LUNCH	
DINNER	
SNACKS	

🏋 EXERCISE

TYPE OF EXERCISE	AMOUNT	NOTES

❤ WELLNESS

I DRANK _____ [CUPS / BOTTLES / OUNCES] OF WATER.

I SLEPT _____ HOURS.

MY MOOD IS _____

_____

I TOOK CARE OF MYSELF BY _____

_____

DATE: _____   WEIGHT: _____

GOAL FOR TODAY

_____

_____

_____

🍎 FOOD

BREAKFAST	
LUNCH	
DINNER	
SNACKS	

🏋 EXERCISE

TYPE OF EXERCISE	AMOUNT	NOTES

❤ WELLNESS

I DRANK _____ [CUPS / BOTTLES / OUNCES] OF WATER.

I SLEPT _____ HOURS.

MY MOOD IS

_____

_____

I TOOK CARE OF MYSELF BY

_____

_____

DATE: _____   WEIGHT: _____

GOAL FOR TODAY

_____
_____
_____

FOOD

BREAKFAST	
LUNCH	
DINNER	
SNACKS	

EXERCISE

TYPE OF EXERCISE	AMOUNT	NOTES

WELLNESS

I DRANK _____ [CUPS / BOTTLES / OUNCES] OF WATER.

I SLEPT _____ HOURS.

MY MOOD IS
_____
_____

I TOOK CARE OF MYSELF BY
_____
_____

Weekly Check-In

Here's your chance to review your progress over the last seven days.

DATE: _____   WEIGHT: _____

MEASUREMENTS

CHEST		THIGHS	
WAIST		CALVES	
HIPS		UPPER ARMS	

OTHER STATS

_____

_____

_____

_____

Are you satisfied with how you did this week in the following areas?
Do you see room for improvement? How?

FOOD
_____

EXERCISE
_____

WATER
_____

SLEEP
_____

SELF-CARE
_____

DATE: _____   WEIGHT: _____

GOAL FOR TODAY

_____

_____

_____

🍎 FOOD

BREAKFAST	
LUNCH	
DINNER	
SNACKS	

EXERCISE

TYPE OF EXERCISE	AMOUNT	NOTES

♡ WELLNESS

I DRANK _____ [CUPS / BOTTLES / OUNCES] OF WATER.

I SLEPT _____ HOURS.

MY MOOD IS _____

_____

I TOOK CARE OF MYSELF BY _____

_____

DATE: _____   WEIGHT: _____

GOAL FOR TODAY

_____

_____

_____

FOOD

BREAKFAST	
LUNCH	
DINNER	
SNACKS	

EXERCISE

TYPE OF EXERCISE	AMOUNT	NOTES

WELLNESS

I DRANK _____ [CUPS / BOTTLES / OUNCES] OF WATER.

I SLEPT _____ HOURS.

MY MOOD IS _____

_____

I TOOK CARE OF MYSELF BY _____

_____

DATE: _____   WEIGHT: _____

GOAL FOR TODAY

_____

_____

_____

FOOD

BREAKFAST	
LUNCH	
DINNER	
SNACKS	

EXERCISE

TYPE OF EXERCISE	AMOUNT	NOTES

WELLNESS

I DRANK _____ [CUPS / BOTTLES / OUNCES] OF WATER.

I SLEPT _____ HOURS.

MY MOOD IS _____

_____

I TOOK CARE OF MYSELF BY _____

_____

DATE: _____   WEIGHT: _____

GOAL FOR TODAY

_____

_____

_____

FOOD

BREAKFAST	
LUNCH	
DINNER	
SNACKS	

EXERCISE

TYPE OF EXERCISE	AMOUNT	NOTES

WELLNESS

I DRANK _____ [CUPS / BOTTLES / OUNCES] OF WATER.

I SLEPT _____ HOURS.

MY MOOD IS _____

_____

I TOOK CARE OF MYSELF BY _____

_____

DATE: _____   WEIGHT: _____

GOAL FOR TODAY

_____

_____

_____

🍎 FOOD

BREAKFAST	
LUNCH	
DINNER	
SNACKS	

🏋 EXERCISE

TYPE OF EXERCISE	AMOUNT	NOTES

💛 WELLNESS

I DRANK _____ [CUPS / BOTTLES / OUNCES] OF WATER.

I SLEPT _____ HOURS.

MY MOOD IS _____

_____

I TOOK CARE OF MYSELF BY _____

_____

DATE: _____   WEIGHT: _____

GOAL FOR TODAY

_____

_____

_____

🍎 FOOD

BREAKFAST	
LUNCH	
DINNER	
SNACKS	

EXERCISE

TYPE OF EXERCISE	AMOUNT	NOTES

♥ WELLNESS

I DRANK _____ [CUPS / BOTTLES / OUNCES] OF WATER.

I SLEPT _____ HOURS.

MY MOOD IS

_____

_____

I TOOK CARE OF MYSELF BY

_____

DATE: _____   WEIGHT: _____

GOAL FOR TODAY

_____
_____
_____

🍎 FOOD

BREAKFAST	
LUNCH	
DINNER	
SNACKS	

🏋 EXERCISE

TYPE OF EXERCISE	AMOUNT	NOTES

❤ WELLNESS

I DRANK _____ [CUPS / BOTTLES / OUNCES] OF WATER.

I SLEPT _____ HOURS.

MY MOOD IS
_____
_____

I TOOK CARE OF MYSELF BY
_____
_____

Weekly Check-In

Here's your chance to review your progress over the last seven days.

DATE: _____ WEIGHT: _____

MEASUREMENTS

CHEST		THIGHS	
WAIST		CALVES	
HIPS		UPPER ARMS	

OTHER STATS

_____

_____

_____

_____

Are you satisfied with how you did this week in the following areas? Do you see room for improvement? How?

FOOD
_____

EXERCISE
_____

WATER
_____

SLEEP
_____

SELF-CARE
_____

DATE: _____   WEIGHT: _____

GOAL FOR TODAY

_____
_____
_____

FOOD

BREAKFAST	
LUNCH	
DINNER	
SNACKS	

EXERCISE

TYPE OF EXERCISE	AMOUNT	NOTES

WELLNESS

I DRANK _____ [CUPS / BOTTLES / OUNCES] OF WATER.

I SLEPT _____ HOURS.

MY MOOD IS
_____
_____

I TOOK CARE OF MYSELF BY
_____
_____

DATE: _____   WEIGHT: _____

GOAL FOR TODAY

_____

_____

_____

FOOD

BREAKFAST	
LUNCH	
DINNER	
SNACKS	

EXERCISE

TYPE OF EXERCISE	AMOUNT	NOTES

WELLNESS

I DRANK _____ [CUPS / BOTTLES / OUNCES] OF WATER.

I SLEPT _____ HOURS.

MY MOOD IS

_____

I TOOK CARE OF MYSELF BY

_____

DATE: _____   WEIGHT: _____

GOAL FOR TODAY

_____

_____

_____

FOOD

BREAKFAST	
LUNCH	
DINNER	
SNACKS	

EXERCISE

TYPE OF EXERCISE	AMOUNT	NOTES

WELLNESS

I DRANK _____ [CUPS / BOTTLES / OUNCES] OF WATER.

I SLEPT _____ HOURS.

MY MOOD IS _____

_____

I TOOK CARE OF MYSELF BY _____

_____

DATE: _____ WEIGHT: _____

GOAL FOR TODAY

_____

_____

_____

🍎 FOOD

BREAKFAST	
LUNCH	
DINNER	
SNACKS	

🏋 EXERCISE

TYPE OF EXERCISE	AMOUNT	NOTES

❤ WELLNESS

I DRANK _____ [CUPS / BOTTLES / OUNCES] OF WATER.

I SLEPT _____ HOURS.

MY MOOD IS _____

_____

I TOOK CARE OF MYSELF BY _____

_____

DATE: _____ WEIGHT: _____

GOAL FOR TODAY

_____

_____

_____

🍎 FOOD

BREAKFAST	
LUNCH	
DINNER	
SNACKS	

EXERCISE

TYPE OF EXERCISE	AMOUNT	NOTES

WELLNESS

I DRANK _____ [CUPS / BOTTLES / OUNCES] OF WATER.

I SLEPT _____ HOURS.

MY MOOD IS _____

_____

I TOOK CARE OF MYSELF BY _____

_____

DATE: _____   WEIGHT: _____

GOAL FOR TODAY

_____

_____

_____

FOOD

BREAKFAST	
LUNCH	
DINNER	
SNACKS	

EXERCISE

TYPE OF EXERCISE	AMOUNT	NOTES

WELLNESS

I DRANK _____ [CUPS / BOTTLES / OUNCES] OF WATER.

I SLEPT _____ HOURS.

MY MOOD IS _____

_____

I TOOK CARE OF MYSELF BY _____

_____

DATE: _____   WEIGHT: _____

GOAL FOR TODAY

_____

_____

_____

🍎 FOOD

BREAKFAST	
LUNCH	
DINNER	
SNACKS	

🏋 EXERCISE

TYPE OF EXERCISE	AMOUNT	NOTES

❤ WELLNESS

I DRANK _____ [CUPS / BOTTLES / OUNCES] OF WATER.

I SLEPT _____ HOURS.

MY MOOD IS _____

_____

I TOOK CARE OF MYSELF BY _____

_____

Weekly Check-In

Here's your chance to review your progress over the last seven days.

DATE: _____   WEIGHT: _____

MEASUREMENTS

CHEST		THIGHS	
WAIST		CALVES	
HIPS		UPPER ARMS	

OTHER STATS

_____

_____

_____

_____

Are you satisfied with how you did this week in the following areas? Do you see room for improvement? How?

FOOD
_____

EXERCISE
_____

WATER
_____

SLEEP
_____

SELF-CARE
_____

DATE: _____   WEIGHT: _____

GOAL FOR TODAY

_____
_____
_____

🍎 FOOD

BREAKFAST	
LUNCH	
DINNER	
SNACKS	

EXERCISE

TYPE OF EXERCISE	AMOUNT	NOTES

WELLNESS

I DRANK _____ [CUPS / BOTTLES / OUNCES] OF WATER.

I SLEPT _____ HOURS.

MY MOOD IS
_____
_____

I TOOK CARE OF MYSELF BY
_____
_____

DATE: _____   WEIGHT: _____

GOAL FOR TODAY

_____

_____

_____

FOOD

BREAKFAST	
LUNCH	
DINNER	
SNACKS	

EXERCISE

TYPE OF EXERCISE	AMOUNT	NOTES

WELLNESS

I DRANK _____ [CUPS / BOTTLES / OUNCES] OF WATER.

I SLEPT _____ HOURS.

MY MOOD IS _____

_____

I TOOK CARE OF MYSELF BY _____

_____

DATE: _____   WEIGHT: _____

GOAL FOR TODAY

_____

_____

_____

FOOD

BREAKFAST	
LUNCH	
DINNER	
SNACKS	

EXERCISE

TYPE OF EXERCISE	AMOUNT	NOTES

WELLNESS

I DRANK _____ [CUPS / BOTTLES / OUNCES] OF WATER.

I SLEPT _____ HOURS.

MY MOOD IS _____

_____

I TOOK CARE OF MYSELF BY _____

_____

DATE: _____ WEIGHT: _____

GOAL FOR TODAY

_____
_____
_____

FOOD

BREAKFAST	
LUNCH	
DINNER	
SNACKS	

EXERCISE

TYPE OF EXERCISE	AMOUNT	NOTES

WELLNESS

I DRANK _____ [CUPS / BOTTLES / OUNCES] OF WATER.

I SLEPT _____ HOURS.

MY MOOD IS _____

_____

I TOOK CARE OF MYSELF BY _____

_____

DATE: _____ WEIGHT: _____

GOAL FOR TODAY

_____
_____
_____

🍎 FOOD

BREAKFAST	
LUNCH	
DINNER	
SNACKS	

EXERCISE

TYPE OF EXERCISE	AMOUNT	NOTES

WELLNESS

I DRANK _____ [CUPS / BOTTLES / OUNCES] OF WATER.

I SLEPT _____ HOURS.

MY MOOD IS _____
_____

I TOOK CARE OF MYSELF BY _____
_____

DATE: _____   WEIGHT: _____

GOAL FOR TODAY

_____

_____

_____

🍎 FOOD

BREAKFAST	
LUNCH	
DINNER	
SNACKS	

🏋 EXERCISE

TYPE OF EXERCISE	AMOUNT	NOTES

❤ WELLNESS

I DRANK _____ [CUPS / BOTTLES / OUNCES] OF WATER.

I SLEPT _____ HOURS.

MY MOOD IS _____

_____

I TOOK CARE OF MYSELF BY _____

_____

DATE: _____   WEIGHT: _____

GOAL FOR TODAY

_____

_____

_____

🍎 FOOD

BREAKFAST	
LUNCH	
DINNER	
SNACKS	

🏋 EXERCISE

TYPE OF EXERCISE	AMOUNT	NOTES

❤ WELLNESS

I DRANK _____ [CUPS / BOTTLES / OUNCES] OF WATER.

I SLEPT _____ HOURS.

MY MOOD IS _____

_____

I TOOK CARE OF MYSELF BY _____

_____

Weekly Check-In

Here's your chance to review your progress over the last seven days.

DATE: _____   WEIGHT: _____

MEASUREMENTS

CHEST		THIGHS	
WAIST		CALVES	
HIPS		UPPER ARMS	

OTHER STATS

_____

_____

_____

_____

Are you satisfied with how you did this week in the following areas? Do you see room for improvement? How?

FOOD
_____

EXERCISE
_____

WATER
_____

SLEEP
_____

SELF-CARE
_____

DATE: _____   WEIGHT: _____

GOAL FOR TODAY

_____

_____

_____

🍎 FOOD

BREAKFAST	
LUNCH	
DINNER	
SNACKS	

🏋 EXERCISE

TYPE OF EXERCISE	AMOUNT	NOTES

❤ WELLNESS

I DRANK _____ [CUPS / BOTTLES / OUNCES] OF WATER.

I SLEPT _____ HOURS.

MY MOOD IS _____

_____

I TOOK CARE OF MYSELF BY _____

_____

DATE: _____ WEIGHT: _____

GOAL FOR TODAY

_____
_____
_____

🍎 FOOD

BREAKFAST	
LUNCH	
DINNER	
SNACKS	

🏋 EXERCISE

TYPE OF EXERCISE	AMOUNT	NOTES

♥ WELLNESS

I DRANK _____ [CUPS / BOTTLES / OUNCES] OF WATER.

I SLEPT _____ HOURS.

MY MOOD IS _____

_____

I TOOK CARE OF MYSELF BY _____

_____

DATE: _____   WEIGHT: _____

GOAL FOR TODAY

_____

_____

_____

FOOD

BREAKFAST	
LUNCH	
DINNER	
SNACKS	

EXERCISE

TYPE OF EXERCISE	AMOUNT	NOTES

WELLNESS

I DRANK _____ [CUPS / BOTTLES / OUNCES] OF WATER.

I SLEPT _____ HOURS.

MY MOOD IS _____

_____

I TOOK CARE OF MYSELF BY _____

_____

DATE: _____   WEIGHT: _____

GOAL FOR TODAY

_____

_____

_____

🍎 FOOD

BREAKFAST	
LUNCH	
DINNER	
SNACKS	

🏋 EXERCISE

TYPE OF EXERCISE	AMOUNT	NOTES

♥ WELLNESS

I DRANK _____ [CUPS / BOTTLES / OUNCES] OF WATER.

I SLEPT _____ HOURS.

MY MOOD IS _____

_____

I TOOK CARE OF MYSELF BY _____

_____

DATE: _____ WEIGHT: _____

GOAL FOR TODAY

_____

_____

_____

FOOD

BREAKFAST	
LUNCH	
DINNER	
SNACKS	

EXERCISE

TYPE OF EXERCISE	AMOUNT	NOTES

WELLNESS

I DRANK _____ [CUPS / BOTTLES / OUNCES] OF WATER.

I SLEPT _____ HOURS.

MY MOOD IS _____

_____

I TOOK CARE OF MYSELF BY _____

_____

DATE: _____   WEIGHT: _____

GOAL FOR TODAY

_____

_____

_____

FOOD

BREAKFAST	
LUNCH	
DINNER	
SNACKS	

EXERCISE

TYPE OF EXERCISE	AMOUNT	NOTES

WELLNESS

I DRANK _____ [CUPS / BOTTLES / OUNCES] OF WATER.

I SLEPT _____ HOURS.

MY MOOD IS _____

_____

I TOOK CARE OF MYSELF BY _____

_____

DATE: _____   WEIGHT: _____

GOAL FOR TODAY

_____

_____

_____

FOOD

BREAKFAST	
LUNCH	
DINNER	
SNACKS	

EXERCISE

TYPE OF EXERCISE	AMOUNT	NOTES

WELLNESS

I DRANK _____ [CUPS / BOTTLES / OUNCES] OF WATER.

I SLEPT _____ HOURS.

MY MOOD IS _____

_____

I TOOK CARE OF MYSELF BY _____

_____

Weekly Check-In

Here's your chance to review your progress over the last seven days.

DATE: _____   WEIGHT: _____

MEASUREMENTS

CHEST		THIGHS	
WAIST		CALVES	
HIPS		UPPER ARMS	

OTHER STATS

_____

_____

_____

Are you satisfied with how you did this week in the following areas?
Do you see room for improvement? How?

FOOD
_____

EXERCISE
_____

WATER
_____

SLEEP

SELF-CARE
_____

DATE: _____   WEIGHT: _____

GOAL FOR TODAY

_____

_____

_____

🍎 FOOD

BREAKFAST	
LUNCH	
DINNER	
SNACKS	

🏋 EXERCISE

TYPE OF EXERCISE	AMOUNT	NOTES

❤ WELLNESS

I DRANK _____ [CUPS / BOTTLES / OUNCES] OF WATER.

I SLEPT _____ HOURS.

MY MOOD IS _____

_____

I TOOK CARE OF MYSELF BY _____

_____

DATE: _____   WEIGHT: _____

GOAL FOR TODAY

_____

_____

_____

FOOD

BREAKFAST	
LUNCH	
DINNER	
SNACKS	

EXERCISE

TYPE OF EXERCISE	AMOUNT	NOTES

WELLNESS

I DRANK _____ [CUPS / BOTTLES / OUNCES] OF WATER.

I SLEPT _____ HOURS.

MY MOOD IS _____

_____

I TOOK CARE OF MYSELF BY _____

_____

DATE: _____   WEIGHT: _____

GOAL FOR TODAY

_____
_____
_____

🍎 FOOD

BREAKFAST	
LUNCH	
DINNER	
SNACKS	

🏋 EXERCISE

TYPE OF EXERCISE	AMOUNT	NOTES

❤ WELLNESS

I DRANK _____ [CUPS / BOTTLES / OUNCES] OF WATER.

I SLEPT _____ HOURS.

MY MOOD IS _____
_____

I TOOK CARE OF MYSELF BY _____
_____

DATE: _____   WEIGHT: _____

GOAL FOR TODAY

_____

_____

_____

🍎 FOOD

BREAKFAST	
LUNCH	
DINNER	
SNACKS	

EXERCISE

TYPE OF EXERCISE	AMOUNT	NOTES

❤ WELLNESS

I DRANK _____ [CUPS / BOTTLES / OUNCES] OF WATER.

I SLEPT _____ HOURS.

MY MOOD IS _____

_____

I TOOK CARE OF MYSELF BY _____

_____

DATE: _____   WEIGHT: _____

GOAL FOR TODAY

_____

_____

_____

FOOD

BREAKFAST	
LUNCH	
DINNER	
SNACKS	

EXERCISE

TYPE OF EXERCISE	AMOUNT	NOTES

WELLNESS

I DRANK _____ [CUPS / BOTTLES / OUNCES] OF WATER.

I SLEPT _____ HOURS.

MY MOOD IS _____

_____

I TOOK CARE OF MYSELF BY _____

_____

DATE: _____   WEIGHT: _____

GOAL FOR TODAY

_____

_____

_____

🍎 FOOD

BREAKFAST	
LUNCH	
DINNER	
SNACKS	

🏋 EXERCISE

TYPE OF EXERCISE	AMOUNT	NOTES

❤ WELLNESS

I DRANK _____ [CUPS / BOTTLES / OUNCES] OF WATER.

I SLEPT _____ HOURS.

MY MOOD IS _____

_____

I TOOK CARE OF MYSELF BY _____

_____

DATE: _____   WEIGHT: _____

GOAL FOR TODAY

_____

_____

_____

🍎 FOOD

BREAKFAST	
LUNCH	
DINNER	
SNACKS	

🏋 EXERCISE

TYPE OF EXERCISE	AMOUNT	NOTES

♥ WELLNESS

I DRANK _____ [CUPS / BOTTLES / OUNCES] OF WATER.

I SLEPT _____ HOURS.

MY MOOD IS _____

_____

I TOOK CARE OF MYSELF BY _____

_____

Weekly Check-In

Here's your chance to review your progress over the last seven days.

DATE: _____   WEIGHT: _____

MEASUREMENTS

CHEST		THIGHS	
WAIST		CALVES	
HIPS		UPPER ARMS	

OTHER STATS

_____

_____

_____

_____

Are you satisfied with how you did this week in the following areas? Do you see room for improvement? How?

FOOD
_____

EXERCISE
_____

WATER
_____

SLEEP
_____

SELF-CARE
_____

DATE: _____   WEIGHT: _____

GOAL FOR TODAY

_____

_____

_____

FOOD

BREAKFAST	
LUNCH	
DINNER	
SNACKS	

EXERCISE

TYPE OF EXERCISE	AMOUNT	NOTES

WELLNESS

I DRANK _____ [CUPS / BOTTLES / OUNCES] OF WATER.

I SLEPT _____ HOURS.

MY MOOD IS _____

_____

I TOOK CARE OF MYSELF BY _____

_____

DATE: _____   WEIGHT: _____

GOAL FOR TODAY

_____

_____

_____

🍎 FOOD

BREAKFAST	
LUNCH	
DINNER	
SNACKS	

🏋 EXERCISE

TYPE OF EXERCISE	AMOUNT	NOTES

❤ WELLNESS

I DRANK _____ [CUPS / BOTTLES / OUNCES] OF WATER.

I SLEPT _____ HOURS.

MY MOOD IS _____

_____

I TOOK CARE OF MYSELF BY _____

_____

DATE: _____   WEIGHT: _____

GOAL FOR TODAY

_____

_____

_____

🍎 FOOD

BREAKFAST	
LUNCH	
DINNER	
SNACKS	

🏋️ EXERCISE

TYPE OF EXERCISE	AMOUNT	NOTES

♥ WELLNESS

I DRANK _____ [CUPS / BOTTLES / OUNCES] OF WATER.

I SLEPT _____ HOURS.

MY MOOD IS _____

_____

I TOOK CARE OF MYSELF BY _____

_____

DATE: _____   WEIGHT: _____

GOAL FOR TODAY

_____

_____

_____

🍎 FOOD

BREAKFAST	
LUNCH	
DINNER	
SNACKS	

🏋 EXERCISE

TYPE OF EXERCISE	AMOUNT	NOTES

❤ WELLNESS

I DRANK _____ [CUPS / BOTTLES / OUNCES] OF WATER.

I SLEPT _____ HOURS.

MY MOOD IS _____

_____

I TOOK CARE OF MYSELF BY _____

_____

DATE: _____   WEIGHT: _____

GOAL FOR TODAY

_____

_____

_____

🍎 FOOD

BREAKFAST	
LUNCH	
DINNER	
SNACKS	

🏋 EXERCISE

TYPE OF EXERCISE	AMOUNT	NOTES

❤ WELLNESS

I DRANK _____ [CUPS / BOTTLES / OUNCES] OF WATER.

I SLEPT _____ HOURS.

MY MOOD IS _____

_____

I TOOK CARE OF MYSELF BY _____

_____

DATE: _____   WEIGHT: _____

GOAL FOR TODAY

_____
_____
_____

FOOD

BREAKFAST	
LUNCH	
DINNER	
SNACKS	

EXERCISE

TYPE OF EXERCISE	AMOUNT	NOTES

WELLNESS

I DRANK _____ [CUPS / BOTTLES / OUNCES] OF WATER.

I SLEPT _____ HOURS.

MY MOOD IS _____

_____

I TOOK CARE OF MYSELF BY _____

_____

DATE: _____   WEIGHT: _____

GOAL FOR TODAY

_____

_____

_____

🍎 FOOD

BREAKFAST	
LUNCH	
DINNER	
SNACKS	

🏋 EXERCISE

TYPE OF EXERCISE	AMOUNT	NOTES

❤ WELLNESS

I DRANK _____ [CUPS / BOTTLES / OUNCES] OF WATER.

I SLEPT _____ HOURS.

MY MOOD IS _____

_____

I TOOK CARE OF MYSELF BY _____

_____

Weekly Check-In

Here's your chance to review your progress over the last seven days.

DATE: _____   WEIGHT: _____

📏 MEASUREMENTS

CHEST		THIGHS	
WAIST		CALVES	
HIPS		UPPER ARMS	

📋 OTHER STATS

_____

_____

_____

_____

Are you satisfied with how you did this week in the following areas?
Do you see room for improvement? How?

FOOD
_____

EXERCISE
_____

WATER
_____

SLEEP
_____

SELF-CARE
_____

DATE: _____   WEIGHT: _____

GOAL FOR TODAY

_____

_____

_____

FOOD

BREAKFAST	
LUNCH	
DINNER	
SNACKS	

EXERCISE

TYPE OF EXERCISE	AMOUNT	NOTES

WELLNESS

I DRANK _____ [CUPS / BOTTLES / OUNCES] OF WATER.

I SLEPT _____ HOURS.

MY MOOD IS _____

_____

I TOOK CARE OF MYSELF BY _____

_____

DATE: _____   WEIGHT: _____

GOAL FOR TODAY

_____
_____
_____

🍎 FOOD

BREAKFAST	
LUNCH	
DINNER	
SNACKS	

EXERCISE

TYPE OF EXERCISE	AMOUNT	NOTES

❤ WELLNESS

I DRANK _____ [CUPS / BOTTLES / OUNCES] OF WATER.

I SLEPT _____ HOURS.

MY MOOD IS _____

_____

I TOOK CARE OF MYSELF BY _____

_____

DATE: _____   WEIGHT: _____

GOAL FOR TODAY

_____
_____
_____

FOOD

BREAKFAST	
LUNCH	
DINNER	
SNACKS	

EXERCISE

TYPE OF EXERCISE	AMOUNT	NOTES

WELLNESS

I DRANK _____ [CUPS / BOTTLES / OUNCES] OF WATER.

I SLEPT _____ HOURS.

MY MOOD IS _____
_____

I TOOK CARE OF MYSELF BY _____
_____

DATE: _____   WEIGHT: _____

GOAL FOR TODAY

_____

_____

_____

FOOD

BREAKFAST	
LUNCH	
DINNER	
SNACKS	

EXERCISE

TYPE OF EXERCISE	AMOUNT	NOTES

WELLNESS

I DRANK _____ [CUPS / BOTTLES / OUNCES] OF WATER.

I SLEPT _____ HOURS.

MY MOOD IS _____

_____

I TOOK CARE OF MYSELF BY _____

_____

DATE: _____ WEIGHT: _____

GOAL FOR TODAY

_____

_____

_____

FOOD

BREAKFAST	
LUNCH	
DINNER	
SNACKS	

EXERCISE

TYPE OF EXERCISE	AMOUNT	NOTES

WELLNESS

I DRANK _____ [CUPS / BOTTLES / OUNCES] OF WATER.

I SLEPT _____ HOURS.

MY MOOD IS _____

_____

I TOOK CARE OF MYSELF BY _____

_____

DATE: _____   WEIGHT: _____

GOAL FOR TODAY

_____

_____

_____

🍎 FOOD

BREAKFAST	
LUNCH	
DINNER	
SNACKS	

EXERCISE

TYPE OF EXERCISE	AMOUNT	NOTES

WELLNESS

I DRANK _____ [CUPS / BOTTLES / OUNCES] OF WATER.

I SLEPT _____ HOURS.

MY MOOD IS _____

_____

I TOOK CARE OF MYSELF BY _____

_____

DATE: _____   WEIGHT: _____

GOAL FOR TODAY

_____
_____
_____

FOOD

BREAKFAST	
LUNCH	
DINNER	
SNACKS	

EXERCISE

TYPE OF EXERCISE	AMOUNT	NOTES

WELLNESS

I DRANK _____ [CUPS / BOTTLES / OUNCES] OF WATER.

I SLEPT _____ HOURS.

MY MOOD IS _____
_____

I TOOK CARE OF MYSELF BY _____
_____

Weekly Check-In

Here's your chance to review your progress over the last seven days.

DATE: _____   WEIGHT: _____

📏 MEASUREMENTS

CHEST		THIGHS	
WAIST		CALVES	
HIPS		UPPER ARMS	

📋 OTHER STATS

_____

_____

_____

_____

Are you satisfied with how you did this week in the following areas? Do you see room for improvement? How?

FOOD
_____

EXERCISE
_____

WATER
_____

SLEEP
_____

SELF-CARE
_____

DATE: _____   WEIGHT: _____

GOAL FOR TODAY

_____
_____
_____

FOOD

BREAKFAST	
LUNCH	
DINNER	
SNACKS	

EXERCISE

TYPE OF EXERCISE	AMOUNT	NOTES

WELLNESS

I DRANK _____ [CUPS / BOTTLES / OUNCES] OF WATER.

I SLEPT _____ HOURS.

MY MOOD IS _____

_____

I TOOK CARE OF MYSELF BY _____

_____

DATE: _____   WEIGHT: _____

GOAL FOR TODAY

_____

_____

_____

FOOD

BREAKFAST	
LUNCH	
DINNER	
SNACKS	

EXERCISE

TYPE OF EXERCISE	AMOUNT	NOTES

WELLNESS

I DRANK _____ [CUPS / BOTTLES / OUNCES] OF WATER.

I SLEPT _____ HOURS.

MY MOOD IS _____

_____

I TOOK CARE OF MYSELF BY _____

_____

DATE: _____   WEIGHT: _____

GOAL FOR TODAY

_____
_____
_____

🍎 FOOD

BREAKFAST	
LUNCH	
DINNER	
SNACKS	

EXERCISE

TYPE OF EXERCISE	AMOUNT	NOTES

♥ WELLNESS

I DRANK _____ [CUPS / BOTTLES / OUNCES] OF WATER.

I SLEPT _____ HOURS.

MY MOOD IS
_____
_____

I TOOK CARE OF MYSELF BY
_____
_____

DATE: _____   WEIGHT: _____

GOAL FOR TODAY

_____
_____
_____

FOOD

BREAKFAST	
LUNCH	
DINNER	
SNACKS	

EXERCISE

TYPE OF EXERCISE	AMOUNT	NOTES

WELLNESS

I DRANK _____ [CUPS / BOTTLES / OUNCES] OF WATER.

I SLEPT _____ HOURS.

MY MOOD IS _____
_____

I TOOK CARE OF MYSELF BY _____
_____

DATE: _____   WEIGHT: _____

GOAL FOR TODAY

_____
_____
_____

🍎 FOOD

BREAKFAST	
LUNCH	
DINNER	
SNACKS	

EXERCISE

TYPE OF EXERCISE	AMOUNT	NOTES

WELLNESS

I DRANK _____ [CUPS / BOTTLES / OUNCES] OF WATER.

I SLEPT _____ HOURS.

MY MOOD IS _____

_____

I TOOK CARE OF MYSELF BY _____

_____

DATE: _____   WEIGHT: _____

GOAL FOR TODAY

_____

_____

_____

FOOD

BREAKFAST	
LUNCH	
DINNER	
SNACKS	

EXERCISE

TYPE OF EXERCISE	AMOUNT	NOTES

WELLNESS

I DRANK _____ [CUPS / BOTTLES / OUNCES] OF WATER.

I SLEPT _____ HOURS.

MY MOOD IS _____

_____

I TOOK CARE OF MYSELF BY _____

_____

DATE: _____   WEIGHT: _____

GOAL FOR TODAY

_____
_____
_____

FOOD

BREAKFAST	
LUNCH	
DINNER	
SNACKS	

EXERCISE

TYPE OF EXERCISE	AMOUNT	NOTES

WELLNESS

I DRANK _____ [CUPS / BOTTLES / OUNCES] OF WATER.

I SLEPT _____ HOURS.

MY MOOD IS _____

_____

I TOOK CARE OF MYSELF BY _____

_____

Weekly Check-In

Here's your chance to review your progress over the last seven days.

DATE: _____   WEIGHT: _____

MEASUREMENTS

CHEST		THIGHS	
WAIST		CALVES	
HIPS		UPPER ARMS	

OTHER STATS

_____

_____

_____

_____

Are you satisfied with how you did this week in the following areas?
Do you see room for improvement? How?

FOOD
_____

EXERCISE
_____

WATER
_____

SLEEP
_____

SELF-CARE
_____

13-Week Check-In

HOW DID YOU DO?

Now's the time to check in on your progress. Fill in the blanks below with today's date. Then go back to page 2 for your original weight and measurements, note them here, and compare the numbers.

DATE: _____

STARTING WEIGHT: _____   CURRENT WEIGHT: _____

MEASUREMENTS

	STARTING	CURRENT
CHEST		
WAIST		
HIPS		
THIGHS		
CALVES		
UPPER ARMS		

OTHER STATS YOU TRACKED

	STARTING	CURRENT

GOALS GOING FORWARD

You've made good progress, so why not make even more? List goals for your next 3 months, and keep training for a healthy life.

THE NEXT 3 MONTHS

WEIGHT: _____

MEASUREMENTS

CHEST	
WAIST	
HIPS	
THIGHS	
CALVES	
UPPER ARMS	

OTHER STATS

NOTES

NOTES

NOTES

NOTES

NOTES